The Ultimate Guide to Enhancing Your Sex Life
For Men & Women
by Tony Xhudo M.S., H.N.
Board Certified by A. A. D. P.

Dedication

This book is dedicated to my lovely wife and life companion,Dawn Xhudo. Who has stood by me through all these years never questioning why, but inspiring me to become the person whom I am today.

Without her inspiration there would be no book, and so I am deeply gratified to have met someone as lovely and devoted as her.

Thank You Hunny For Being There For When I've Needed You Most To Be !!!   "I Love You"

TABLE OF CONTENTS

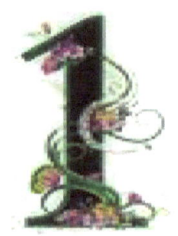

CHAPTER ONE

<u>Sex and Health</u>

"Sex alleviates tension. Love causes it." – WOODY ALLEN

Much has been said about the wonders and pleasure's of sex through the ages. Sex, something that is thought about in both men and women on a daily basis. It is said that 85% of most men in their 20 to 30's think about sex every 52 seconds or so. Women the same age only think about sex once a day, except during the time of ovulation when its three to four times during the day.

In this book we will discover that there should be no reason why anyone regardless of age should be able to enjoy and experience the pleasure's of sexual fulfillment. We will find out how to obtain a healthy libido in both sexes through diet, vitamins/minerals, herbs, and prescription drugs. Also discovering why so many at an early age fail to perform sexually. Uncovering hidden undiagnosed health problems concerning sexual dysfunction.

In Pfizer's 2007 Global Study of Sexual Attitudes and Behaviors, 64 percent of women (ages 40 to 80) in 28 countries felt that sex was an important part of their lives, and that physical and sexual satisfaction were highly correlated with feeling healthy and happy. Nearly 70 percent of those who described their health as "excellent" also reported that their physical relationship with their partner was extremely pleasurable. As you can see sex even as we get in our older years is important in our society.

In my 20 years of practice as a holistic health practitioner, I've successfully helped thousands of men and women restore (and/or balance) their libido. I have learned that with trial and error, helping men and woman achieve better sexual health is not only possible, but easily attainable!

Men in the sexual department certainly have an edge, with drugs such as Viagra, Levitra, and Cialis. As of the current moment Big Pharma is in the process of trying to produce a female version of Viagra.

In today's society we are fortunate with so many available solutions about sex, whether they come from natural sources or pharmaceutically.

This search in sexual enhancement has led to the development of pills and understanding of how certain neurotransmitter's dopamine,and serotonin and testosterone's affect our sexual behavior in both men and women which can help enhance libido and sexual dysfunction. Through out this book you will understand how sexual enhancing nutrients and drugs affect our brain's neurotransmitter's. You will learn how our hormones and neurotransmitters govern our desire and sex drive,and find the right prescription for our sexual moods.

CHAPTER TWO

<u>Oxytocin The Hormone of Love & Bonding</u>

"The good thing about masturbation is that you don't have to get dressed up for it" - Truman Capote

The act of sex has many health benefits that helps promote longevity and happiness. Sexual satisfaction helps establish a positive relationship in those with monamagus relationships. Just the mere touch and a caress from a female partner helps produce oxytocin, the chemical of love. Oxytocin, secreted by the brain's pituitary gland is what bonds us together, it's what's released everytime we give or receive hugs or having orgasms in both sexes. Has been described as the hormone of motherly love,the hormone of monogamy and the equivalent to super glue as it is important for binding relationships together.

The levels of oxytocin also rise everytime we tend to think of someone your fond of and surge higher when you are in close proximity to touch them. Having sex will send oxytocin levels soaring to five times than the normal level.

In the brain, oxytocin is involved in social recognition and bonding,and may also be involved in the formation of trust between two people. In women its released in large amounts during labor and child birth and in nipple stimulation during breastfeeding. Dr. Teresa Crenshaw defines the power of touch as

"Vitamin T".

 Through caressing, hugging, stroking, and cuddling, the body releases a chain reaction of chemicals that sends a signal to your brain that what you are experiencing is pleasurable, assuring and good. MDMA (ecstasy) a love drug may increase feelings of love, empathy and connection to others by stimulating oxytocin activity via activation of serotonin 5-HT1A receptors.

From an emotional point of view,the rise of oxytocin levels that occur with skin to skin contact and at the point of climax helps you and your partner bind that much closer but will also make you feel drowsy so you enjoy an even more refreshing and restorative night's sleep after making love. As you can see, oxytocin has the ability to influence us in so many positive ways. There are many commercial products which can be found on the internet that helps to raise your oxytocin levels by means of a spray called "Liquid Trust" that you spray on your body or clothing that actually contains "oxytocin" and has a 100% money back guarantee.

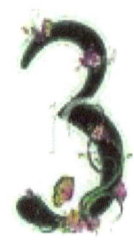

CHAPTER THREE

<u>Dopamine -The Feel Good Chemical of Love & Desire</u>

Dopamine is the brain's pleasure chemical (a monoamine neurotransmitter) that drives the desire and anticipation for pleasure. It plays a very important part in the brain system that is responsible for a reward driven learning response, sex, food, drugs, pleasure, addiction's, depression, happiness, feelings of enjoyment, motor control (Parkison's, lack of dopamine) regulates prolactin, social behavoir, and sexual pleasures.

We can fill this entire book about research articles and sexual function on just dopamine but we'll just focus on the importance of sexual function and libido. Dopamine is the central player when it comes to sexual desire, erections, sex fetishes, and sexual addictions. One of the most common complaints is erectile dysfunction,which is due to an over stimulation of the reward system circuitry. Over stimulation of dopamine leads to a reduction of dopamine receptors (D2) which are necessary for erections.

Testosterone increases sexual desire by stimulating dopamine in the brain. Sexual satiety leads to fewer testosterone receptors, thus less dopamine. Sexual function doesn't correlate with blood levels of testosterone but there is more evidence that testosterone affects libido and erections by facilitating dopamine. We know that testosterone and dopamine are tightly inter linked,as anything that raises testosterone or adrenaline in the body will also raise dopamine levels.

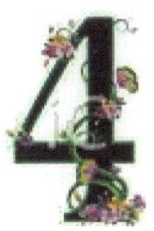

CHAPTER FOUR

<u>Stress & Libido</u>

In today's society there are many physiological factors that affect dopamine. Stress,life style,bad dieting,over weight and lack of exercise, can all contribute to low levels of testosterone and dopamine. Stress is thee most common cause of low libido,along with overwork,tiredness and a lack of sleep. When under extreme stress the adrenal glands produce an increased amount of cortisol and adrenaline instead,and the adrenal boost to sex drive switches off. The adrenal glands produce about 5% of the circulating sex hormones such as estrogen and testosterone.

Stress will significantly reduce levels of DHEA in the brain and also decrease the secretions of gonadotrophin releasing hormone (GnRH) the master hormone that kicks in the ovaries and testicles to start producing oestrogen and testosterone. One of the most tell tale causes of reduced sex drive in stressed individuals is increased levels of the hormone prolactin which occurs in surges in times of stress to turn off the sex drive. This is also one of the most common associated problems in sexual dysfunction.

Reducing levels of stress will help to boost sex drive in both men and women. Relaxation techniques followed by a whole food diet and exercise will often produce miraculous results in your well being and libido. So by controlling cortisol and managing the triggers of stress is the key to hormonal balance and over all health.

Supplements and Stress Control

At times of difficulties in managing our life style, we can help ourselves by supplementing our diet with certain nutrients and herbs to counter the stress levels at hand. Sometimes dietary changes is all that it is needed to restore libido and refuel our desires. Like a lack of essential fatty acids,as well as a protein deficient diet,may inhibit neural stimulation,thus contributing to sexual apathy. Supplementing with **DHEA** (a hormone naturally produced by the adrenal glands) may increase libido in some women. As we age,the body's production of DHEA declines gradually,and according to Beth M. Ley in her book DHEA:Unlocking the Secrets to the Fountain of Youth,she notes that studies indicate that supplementing with DHEA can improve one's sex drive and increase fertility.

DHEA can also benefit you in stress reduction. You would be better suited to supplement with **Pregnenlone**, which is made by the body from cholesterol. Pregnenlone is the basic precursor to the starting raw material for the production of all the body's steroidal hormones, including DHEA, progesterone, estrogen, testosterone, cortisol and Aldosterone and as such is often referred to as the mother of all hormones.

Pregnenlone is also becoming to be a very popular anti-aging hormone by so many ant-aging enthusiasts. Pregnenlone has been studied and used extensively since as early as 1930's. Experiments that were once conducted in the 1940's and 1950's found that Pregnenlone increases productivity and reduced the stress of factory workers.

As an excellent anti-inflammatory in conditions as, arthritis and allergies, Pregnenlone was soon to be phased out of medical use. Ironically is much more safer and versatile than certain specific steroidal hormones that later on replaced it,obviously a political move made by big pharmaceutical drug companies to abolish a natural product that they could not patent. For stress control Pregnelone is my first choice as it blocks out the effects of Cortisol. But like DHEA Pregnenlone also declines with age and supplementation with this supplement will bring about many positive benefits to your over all well being and health.

Because Pregnenlone can enhance DHEA levels some do believe it would benefit to take both and make for a perfect companion to DHEA. According to biochemist Raymond Peat PhD, who has taken and experiment with Pregnenlone for many years feels that it will benefit the human body in stress reduction,mind enhancement,cognitive function,improve memory,relieve depression,anti-inflammatory response,and most important reduce stress induced fatigue.

As you can see Pregnenlone will be of benefit and an important supplement to consider for improved moods and sexual well being. Pregnenlone is most effective when taken in the morning hours before eating. Some physicians recommend starting out with just 5mgs. Daily unless you are older or are taking it for a special condition in which case you can try and take 30-60mgs. But a typical recommendation is between 5mgs and 30 mgs per day. I myself take,along with my wife take 50mgs per day every morning Monday thru Fridays only with Saturday and Sunday being a break as to let the body manufacture some of its own.

Effective Herbal Remedies For Stress Control and Sex Drive

The wonders of nature always seem to amaze me when it comes to finding a remedy for what ever ails us. Way before drug companies were ever in existence, herbs were the medicine of choice throughout the world. Chinese Herbology dates as far back as 4,000 years ago and Ayurverdic (Indian) goes back even further 6,000 years ago.

An interesting herb of value when it comes to stress management and sex enhancement is an herb called Rhodiola Rosea, also called Aron's Rod or Golden Root. This herb is primarily found in the colder regions of the rocky mountains of Russia, The Alps, Scandinavia, and Central Asia. For years the people in those geographic areas have used the herb to stave off the cold and physical stress of the harsh environment in which they lived in.

The health properties of Rhodiola Rosea contains various compounds that are believed to work together to optimize levels of certain brain neurotransmitters of dopamine and serotonin,and you can see that as we spoke of dopamine in earlier chapters of how it effects sexuality. The root of this herb is classified as an Adaptogen which can increase sexual potency and physical endurance and Adaptogens are natural plant substances that increases the body's resistance and normalize the functions of the body when a stressful situation occurs. Adaptogens allow our body to handle the stressful situation's in a more resourceful state.

Rhodiola Rosea supplements usually come in capsule or tablet form which should be taken in the early morning hours during the first few weeks as it can cause insomnia. This herb works best when taken on an empty stomach about a half hour before breakfast. Dosage's should be about 50mgs and no more than 200 mgs. This herb is also reportedly to work well with Valerian Root and St. John's Wort.

According to Dr. Mehmet Oz, director at the Cardiovascular Institute, New York Presbyterian/Columbia, this herb can actually help improve prostate function and erectile dysfunction. In his book "Medicine Hunter" author Chris Kilham states Rhodiola Rosea does have sexual enhancement properties.

In today's market of sex pills and aphrodisiacs there are so many commercial products available for sale and to know what works and what doesn't tends to be expensive and time consuming. It is estimated that 40% of women complain of poor libido in some point of their lives and women compared to men are more likely to experience poor sex drive. Not to say that men don't have their fair share of them either.

Generally speaking I believe that lifestyle changes like exercise and diet focused on foods and nutrients that increase brain chemistry are the first step in restoring health and alleviating any sexual disorders. It all begins in the brain.

-

CHAPTER FIVE

Foods For Great Sex

There are specific foods that can be eaten to give one a sexual boost foods like, bananas, carrots, asparagus, mandrake, magnosteen, cacao, walnuts, almonds, ginseng, cucumbers, oysters, calms, figs, celery, wild yams, cabbage, and garlic just to name a few.

Asparagus – Contains Vitamin E stimulates hormone production and adrenal sex hormones.

Celery- Contains the hormone Androsterone, an orderless male hormone that's know to turn women on.

Garlic – Very good for circulation and helps with the production of testosterone.

Oysters – High in Zinc a mineral that's required for the production of Testosterone and also thought to contain Dopamine.

Figs – High in Amino Acids are thought to increase libido and sexual stamina.

Wild Yams – Contains precursors thought to aid in the production of the body's natural steroidal hormones.

Walnuts- Contains essential fatty acids necessary for hormone production.

Almonds – Helps with testosterone production and high in amino acids.

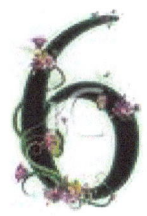

CHAPTER SIX

<u>Sex and Brain Chemistry</u>

A decrease in sexual interest may be the first indicator that there is a problem within four of the brain chemicals Dopamine, Acetylcholine, Gaba, and Serotonin. We will look into each one and see how it corresponds to sexual function.

Acetylcholine – When we have too much of this neurotransmitter we lubricate very easily and feel romantic. We're intuitive and always looking for new problems to solve. Our cognitive levels improve,our thinking process doubles erections become more attainable orgasms become more pleasurable and feels of romance intensifies.

Signs of Low Levels of Acetylcholine - Not being turned on by touch or massage ,miss interpreting people's emotions, dry or cracked skin, poor memory, cognitive decline, poor erections, poor vaginal lubrication, poor arousal response in both men and women.

Dopamine – High levels are associated with high sex drive in both men and women,physically attracted to the opposite sex. Sexual senses are more attuned addictions to sex, porn, gambling, drug use, and nicotine.

Dopamine & Low levels – with low levels of Dopamine your libido is low, your erections are weak, with women orgasms become weak, sexual frequency drops and basically you lose your sexually fire.

The central job of Dopamine is to keep us working and motivated towards our lifestyle. Engaged in activities such as sex, eating, making one feel good with the task at hand. A Dopamine deficiency may also be affecting your Cortisol levels,for every brain chemical that becomes deficient there's another one to take its place. The body will naturally increase the production cortisol when there is a Dopamine imbalance,because the body will use cortisol as a back up energy hormone. Providing us with the additional required to function and be happy.

When Dopamine is being replaced by Cortisol you may not be aware that you are low in Dopamine. You will continue to feel happy and energetic until it completely comes to a stop and realize that your blood pressure is up, you've become bloated, puffy looking in the face,unable to sleep at night, weight gained especially around the abdomen becomes abnormally noticeable, having a hard time waking up and feeling refreshed.

In fact when you are stressed your body naturally releases Cortisol whether or not your Dopamine levels are low or not and you will also burn more Dopamine causing the release of more Cortisol production.

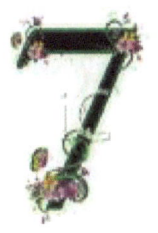

CHAPTER SEVEN

<u>FOODS & DOPAMINE</u>

The easiest way to build up more Dopamine and increase your sex life is through food. These foods contain Amino Acids and proteins that are precursors to Dopamine. If you are deficient in Dopamine you would want to focus on foods rich in the amino acid **L-Tyrosine and L-Phenylaline**. Both of these amino acids are high in protein foods, such as meats and poultry, dairy products and wheat germ. The Amino Acid Tyrosine is also a natural stress fighter and acts as a natural pain reliever as well.

<u>Foods That Create Dopamine</u>

- *Bananas*
- *Wild Game*
- *Cottage Cheese*
- *Pork*
- *Poultry*
- *Wheat Germ*
- *Walnuts*
- *Almonds*
- *Lean Beef*
- *Eggs*

- *Yogurt*
- *Soy Products*

Mucuna Puriens (L-Dopa) – A herb which contains significant amounts of L-Dopa that readily converts into Dopamine, look for the highest percentage extract.

Ginkgo Biloba - An Extraordinary herb that can increase blood supple to the brain and increase's dopamine levels. Make sure it standardized for 24% Ginkgolides and Flavanoids. In Europe used as a treatment for dementia.

L-Tyrosine – Precursor to dopamine production. Helps also to support thyroid function and is excellent for stress & fatigue.

L-Phenylalanine- converts into L-Tyrosine which converts into dopamine. Has been used for pain management as well.

Rhodiola Rosea – Balances serotonin and dopamine levels and helps reduce and balance excessive levels of cortisol.

Thiamine,B1 – Increases dopamine levels in the brain.

NADH – A Coenzyme that is found in all living cells and has been used in Alzheimer's and Parkinson's patients. Besides that it enhances brain levels of dopamine it also helps with cognitive related functions of the brain, memory, learning, depression, concentration, learning and energy part of the Krebs cycle of ATP production.

SAM e – (S-adenosylmethionine) Is an amino acid derivative that's normally synthesized in the body and concentrated in the brain and liver. It is a methyl donor in the synthesis of hormones, neurotransmitters, nucleic acids, proteins,and phospholids and catecholamines, and the neuro transmitters dopamine and serotonin. SAM e is required for the synthesis of nor ephinephrine, dopamine and serotonin. In 2002, the U.S. Department of Health and Human Services conducted a meticulous evaluation of SAM e showing its findings the efficacy of SAM e in helping to maintain and improve joint function stability without any related side effects.

Vitamin B6- needed in the metabolism of dopamine and metabolism of most amino acid's.

N-Acetyl-L-Tyrosine – More of a bio-available form of Tyrosine that's readily absorbed and helps to raise levels of Dopamine.

L-Thea-nine – Helps to balance levels of Serotonin and Dopamine, and counter the effects of stress related Cortisol.

Green Tea – Affects Dopamine release, and for a double dose of Dopamine pleasure try steeping two tea bags of green tea in a cup of hot water and add a pinch of cayenne powder. Contains high concentrations of L-Thea-nine .

Citicoline – Studies suggest that CPD-choline supplements improve dopamine receptor densities that can help improve memory and concentration, and may be useful in the treatment of attention deficient disorder's.

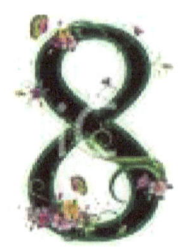

CHAPTER EIGHT

<u>Smart Drugs & Pharmaceuticals that Increase Dopamine Levels</u>

Cocaine – A recreational drug that raise dopamine levels rapidly. An alkaloid that comes from the leaves of the coca plant and a potent central nervous stimulant that produces a euphoric sense of happiness and energy. As you can see from its popularity that it can intensify sexual feelings and stimulation can be amplified from the dopamine release.

Marijuana – Another recreational drug used in mind alterations contains the chemical THC which affects the brain's level of dopamine and nor epinephrine that influences mood and behavior.

Methamphetamine's – A psycho stimulant that's also been abused and is becoming very popular amongst the young crowd of individuals. When methamphetamine's enter the brain they provide a cascade of neurotransmitter release of serotonin,nor epinephrine,and dopamine release. Since it stimulates the brain's reward center pathways it produces a euphoric sense of excitement leading to its widespread addiction.

Ecstasy (MDMA) – another popular recreational sex drug that is commonly found and distributed in clubs through out the country. Its affect on the brain and the body are rather complex it induces Serotonin, Dopamine,and Nor-ephinephrine release and several hormones including Prolactin, Oxycontin, ACTH, DHEA, and the anti-diuretic hormone Vasopressin. The effects are quite dramatic and produce a mental sense of euphoria and happiness, increased feelings of empathy and closeness, a heightened sense of touch, increased sense of social ability, increased sense of urge to communicate with others, and the list goes on.

It doesn't come without its side effects, such as increased blood pressure, and heart rate,increased body temperature,jaw clenching (bruximia) and in males possible erection dysfunction.

Nicotine – Activates the same reward neural pathways in the brain that other drugs do as Cocaine and Amphetamines do. Research does show that nicotine increases Dopamine levels in the brain and as you can see the chasing the tail effect. The pleasure of each cigarette consumed wears off within minutes and hence the addiction side of cigarette's, reward seeking effect of pleasure Dopamine. People must continue dosing themselves with nicotine to satisfy their addiction related high. But there are other alternatives in this book as you can see and read on.

Wellbutrin- An anti-depressant that enhances the availability of Dopamine in the brain, and increases sexual desire in men and women. A study in 2009 in the Journal of Sex and Marital Therapy reported that nearly one-third of the participants who were on Wellbutrin reported more sexual desire and fantasy about sexual encounters.

Adderall & Ritalin – Amphetamines that can enhance levels of dopamine and Nor-epineephrine levels of the body.

Deprenyl & Eldepryl – May increase sexual desire's in men and women by enhance levels of dopamine. Commonly used to treat Parkinson's depression and dementia a very popular anti aging drug used by many in the life extention.

Cabergoline (Dostinex) – A powerful Dopamine agnostic that lowers prolactin levels successfully. For management in Hyperprolactemia and its symptoms, Dostinex is the drug of choice in the terms of effectiveness and undesirable side effects. It does this very well in both men and women and since it gets rid of Orolactin so successfully it will even resolve sexual dysfunction. Life extentionist are also very big on this drug as a Dopamine agnostic it helps to control the flow of information in the brain. But concerning Dopamine and sex, it's the drug of choice that is a favorite amongst many. Dostinex will improve libido, ejaculation, orgasmic response, refractory response between love making. The positives are many with Dostinex and side effects are few. This is one drug of choice that's worth remembering about.

Bromocriptine (Parlodel) – Another Dopamine agnostic similar to Dostinex and similar in function. But not quite as powerful as Dostinex. The effects as a sexual drug are the same but side effects are more pronounced. Also used in Parkinson's and female infertility and in Hyperprolactemia.

Apomorphine (Uprima) - Used to treat Parkinson's disorder that comes in a solution that's injected subcutaneously just under the skin that comes in a glass cartridge with an injection pen or derivative of morphine that is extracted from opium but not quite as strong as a flavored medication that dissolves under the tongue. Apomorphine works by triggering certain area's of the brain in the hypothalamus that increases the production of dopamine. Used in Europe to treat male impotence. Uprima has a strong effect in enducing erections that goes to work rather quickly,because it dissolves rapidly by passing the digestive tract and going into the blood stream quickly within 15 minutes or so. In one study over 60 patients living with impotence admitted that they experienced a vast improvement in sexual function and activity in the ten week trial. Not yet approved for in the united states for erectile dysfunction but readily used in Europe and was the first oral therapy to be approved for the treatment of erectile dysfunction by the European Commission for the treatment of ED.

Modafinil – used to treat narcolepsy but increasingly used to enhance cognitive abilities by affecting the activity of dopamine in the brain that may create the potential for abuse and dependance ,according to the study done by JAMA. Modafinil is also used in off label use in cognitive dysfunction in some psychiatric disorders i.e. ADHD,and Schizophrenia. We have to bare in mind that all Dopaminergic drugs do have the potential for abuse and one should seek the help of a qualified practitioner of medicine or a pharmacologist.

As you can see how dopamine affects pleasure and addiction that plays a crucial role in our mental health and sexuality. By increasing the amount

Dopamine in certain regions of the brain that give rise to sexual pleasure's and stimulation, we can potentiate it's effects through diet, supplements and drugs. Many of these products do have different effects on men and women,and you must be cautious as just like anything else do have side effects that can positive and some negative.

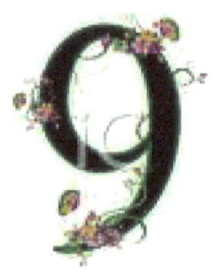

CHAPTER NINE

<u>The Role of Serotonin and Sexual Function</u>

Serotonin a neurotransmitter and neuro-hormone that regulates functions through out the body sending signals between nerve cells that alters brain chemistry to adjust mood, behavior, sexual function,and sleep. It's also the only neurotransmitter that's classified as a neuro-hormone as well,and has a powerful affect on our moods and behavior. When your serotonin levels are high you will experience headaches, agitation, confusion, and restlessness. When they are low we experience depression, severe anxiety, panic disorder, and OCD (*obsessive compulsive disorder*). As far as sexual behavior is concerned,serotonin keeps the joy in sexual relationships by allowing us to feel pleasure and to feel good about ourselves. Adequate levels of serotonin are important for appetite control, memory recall, deep restful sleep, and a host of feel good chemicals to experience sex.

If your levels drop you will likely fall into a depression,become irritable,angry,and for some people become suicidal. It is evident that serotonin is an extremely important neurotransmitter that has a multitude of bodily processes and brain functions. As it pertains to sexual function,too little serotonin may be the cause of premature ejaculation since serotonin in the brain is one of the molecules involved in ejaculation. On the opposite end too much serotonin will cause orgasms without an erection. Women on the other hand with very high levels of serotonin can experience prolonged delays in orgasms and the need for their partner to extend sexual stimulation in order to have an orgasm.

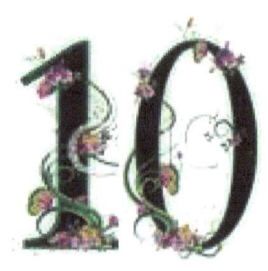

CHAPTER TEN

<u>Natural Alternatives To Increasing Serotonin Levels With Smart Drugs & Pharmaceuticals</u>

<u>Foods</u>

Bananas   **Chicken**   **Nuts**

Turkey   **Soy**   **Cottage Cheese**

Milk (especially warm-to-hot)   **Soy Milk**

Beans   **Eggs**   **Rice**

Seafood   **Peanuts Lentils   Oats**

Whole Grains   Sweet Potato

Beef Spinach   Tuna Halibut

Shrimp   Snapper   Sun Flower Seeds

Spirulina   Pumkin   Squash

Flaxseed   Mushrooms   Turnip Greens

Natural Supplements

Tryptophan - An amino acid that's the serves as a precursor to serotonin,and because of its ability to raise levels of serotonin it has been used extensively in therapeutic conditions as, OCD, anxiety disorders, sleep disorder's, insomnia, panic attacks, phobias and depression. Regarded as an essential amino acid and very important to our daily diet for growth and mental functioning that without it humans could not survive. Tryptophan comes in 500mg. Capsules and can be purchased at any health food store. The dosage may vary for some,from 500mgs to 1,500mgs taken several times a day on an empty stomach always as it will compete for absorbtion with other amino acid's if taken with food. It Also helps when taken Tryptophan to also take it with vitamin B6 and vitamin c,which help with the metabolism of Tryptophan in its conversion to serotonin. Other co-factors that help in the metabolism of serotonin, are folic acid and magnesium.

5-HTP - 5 Hydroxy-Tryptophan which is the conversion of Tryptophan to 5-HTP in the immediate form that converts into serotonin ,can also be purchased in supplement form and comes in 50mgs to 100mgs strength's. Dosages vary from 50mgs to 200mgs depending on the condition being taken for.

St. John's Wart – (*Hypericum Perforatum*) one of the most common herbs used for emotional disorders that appears to have antidepressant activity. With the two active compounds being Hypericin and Hyperforin, which may affect the brains serotonin system. In some of the research past studies it was determined to be more effective than the prescription antidepressant (Zoloft) and (Prozac) but not a placebo.

Amongst the emotional disorders St. John's Wort was determined to effective were, OCD, anxiety, depression, and in other area's of non-emotional disorders were, skin conditions, ear pain, smoking cessation, menopausal symptoms and seasonal affective disorder. Side effects noted in recent studies were associated with short term use of St. John's Wort were, mild stomach upset, allergic skin reactions, restlessness, sexual/erectile dysfunction, dizziness, dry mouth, and tiredness. St.John's Wort should also not taken with certain drugs,medications,and alcohol as it may interact and be potentially harmful. Also note that the supplement "iron" blocks the absorption of St. John's Wort. All in all St. John's Wort is a relatively safe herb that's been used by many successfully for generations,but caution is always still advised when it comes to use of herb's.

Vitamin B6 (*Pyridoxine*) – mainly responsible for the production and metabolism of neurotransmitters, serotonin, melatonin, dopamine,nor-epinephrine, and Gaba. Vitamin B6 is responsible for the processing of amino acids and proteins. It can be found naturally in a variety of foods including red meats, poultry, fish, eggs, non-citrus foods, and cereals.

The optimum intake is yet known but the typical dosage range is 2-20 mgs a day although in can be purchased in varying dosage's 50 to 100mgs.

Folic Acid & Vitamin C – play a role in the production of serotonin and transmitting brain chemicals.

Sun Light – bright sunlight increases the production of serotonin in the body and also bright lights,so spend some time in the sun for the serotonin enhancing effect.

Meditation – this helps the nervous system operate at optimum levels,increasing levels of serotonin and endorphins.

Exercise – one of the best natural ways to increase levels of serotonin and endorphins. Try training vigorously for 45 minutes or so ,putting a physical demand on the body to stimulate the effects of serotonin and endorphins. Everyone, I'm sure at one time or another has felt the soothing calm effects after exercising, whether it be long distance jogging, running, tennis, weightlifting, or even playing basketball.

Pharmaceutical's and Drug's that Enhance Serotonin Levels

Prozac – *(Fluoxetine)* *- is a class of pharmaceutical drug's called selective re-uptake inhibitors (SSRI) that was the first approved (SSRI) drug by FDA in 1987 is used for major depression, OCD, extreme anxiety, generalized socialized anxiety disorders, and panic attacks. Prozac was the drug of choice prescribed by many physicians during its marketing introduc*tion hype in main stream medicine. Prozac works by adjusting serotonin levels in the brain by preventing the re-uptake of serotonin by nerve cells after its been released.

Since uptake is an important mechanism for removing released neurotransmitters and terminating their actions on adjacent nerves the reduced uptake then increases free serotonin levels to stimulate nerve cells in the brain. The side effects that have been reported of Prozac are sexual dysfunction in both man and women patients, low sex drive, dry mouth, anger issues, decreased appetite, and headaches.

Paxil (*Paroxitine*) – an antidepressant that's listed as a serotonin re-uptake inhibitor that affects brain chemicals that may be unbalanced. Paxil is also used to similar situations as Prozac and also may be used for additional purposes such as, severe premenstrual disorder, premature ejaculation in men, and the nerve problems that are associated with diabetic neuropathy.

Paxil as in all (SSRI's) drugs should be used with caution and should not be mixed with any other drugs or medicine's

Lithium – An element that's found in trace amounts in virtually all rocks. Lithiun works with other elements in the brain by increasing serotonin release and decreasing serotonin receptors in the hypothalamus. Lithium is currently the most commonly used drug to treat bi-polar disorders. It serves as a mood stabilizer and is helpful in 70% to 80 % in bipolar patients.

Zoloft -   (*Sertraline HCI*) also belongs to a class of drugs called (SSRI's) serotonin re uptake inhibitors that's used in OCD,panic disorders,anxiety,major depression,post traumatic stress disorder,and premenstrual dysphoric disorder. Side effects are the same as with other (SSRI's) class drugs, low sex drive, sexual dysfunction, etc.

These are just some of the pharmaceutical drugs currently out pertaining to serotonin re uptake inhibitors. There are many more which basically cover what I've mentioned and they all pertain to the same common emotional disorders listed in the previous pages. Some people do well on certain listed drugs and for some people it's a matter of trial and error to see what works. You have to remember that we are all biologically the same but sometimes the same drug will have different effects on certain individuals.

The sexual dysfunction that some of these serotonin drugs may cause will have a different affect opposite of what's mostly commonly experienced. This is why scientists today still regard the brain as very complex and not yet fully understood.

CHAPTER ELEVEN

<u>The Role of Serotonin and Sexual Function</u>

Serotonin a neurotransmitter and neurohormone that regulates functions through out the body sending signals between nerve cells that alters brain chemistry to adjust mood, behavior, sexual function, and sleep. Its also the only neurotransmitter that's classified as a neurohormone as well,and has a powerful affect on our moods and behavior. When your serotonin levels are high

you will experience headaches,agitation,confusion,and restlessness. When they are low we experience depression, severe anxiety, panic disorder, and

OCD -obsessive complusive disorder. As far as sexual behavior is concerned serotonin keeps the joy in sexual relationships by allowing us to feel pleasure and to feel good about ourselves. Adequate levels of serotonin are important for appetite control, memory recall, deep restful sleep, and a host of feel good chemicals to experience sex.

If your levels drop you will likely fall into a depression, become irritable, angry, and for some people become suicidal. It is evident that serotonin is an extremely important neurotransmitter that has a multitude of bodily processes and brain functions. As it pertains to sexual function, too little serotonin may be the cause of premature ejaculation since serotonin in the brain is one of the molecules involved in ejaculation. On the opposite of end, too much serotonin will cause orgasms without an erection. Women on the other hand with very high levels of serotonin can experience prolonged delays in orgasms and the need for their partner to extend sexual stimulation in order to have an orgasm.

Natural Alternatives To Increasing Serotonin Levels With Smart Drugs & Pharmaceuticals

Foods

- **Bananas**
- **Chicken**
- **Nuts**
- **Turkey**
- **Soy**
- **Cottage Cheese**

- **Milk (especially warm-to-hot)**
- **Soy Milk**
- **Beans**
- **Eggs**
- **Rice**

- **Seafood**
- **Peanuts**
- **Lentils**
- **Oats**

- **Whole Grains**
- **Sweet Potato**
- **Beef**
- **Spinach**
- **Tuna**
- **Halibut**
- **Shrimp**
- **Snapper**
- **Sun Flower Seeds**
- **Spirulina**
- **Pumkin**
- **Squash**
- **Flaxseed**
- **Mushrooms**
- **Turnip Greens**

Natural Supplements

Tryptophan - An amino acid that serves as a precursor to serotonin, and because of its ability to raise levels of serotonin it has been used extensively in therapeutic conditions such as OCD, anxiety disorders, sleep disorders, insomnia, panic attacks, phobias, and depression. Regarded as an essential amino acid and very important to our daily diet for growth and mental functioning. Without it humans could not survive. Tryptophan comes in 500mg. Capsules and can be purchased at any health food store. The dosage may vary for some, from 500 mgs to 1,500 mgs taken several times a day on an empty stomach always as it will compete for absorption with other amino acids if taken with food. It Also helps when taken Tryptophan to also take it with vitamin B6 and Vitamin C which help with the metabolism of Tryptophan in its conversion to serotonin. Other co-factors that help in the metabolism of serotonin are Folic Acid and Magnesium.

5-HTP - (*5-hydroxy-tryptophan*) Is the conversion of tryptophan to 5-HTP in the immediate form that converts into serotonin can also be purchased in supplement form and comes in 50mgs to 100mgs strengths. Dosages vary from 50mgs to 200mgs depending on the condition being taken for.

St.John's Wart – (*Hypericum Perforatum*) One of the most common herbs used for emotional disorders that appears to have anti deppressant activity. With the two active compounds being hypericin and hyperforin which may affect the brains serotonin system. In some of the research past studies it was determined to be more effective than the prescription antidepressant (Zoloft) and (Prozac) but not a placebo.

Amongst the emotional disorders St. John's Wort was determined to be effective for OCD, anxiety, depression, and in other area's of non-emotional disorders were skin conditions, ear pain, smoking cessation, menopausal symptoms, and seasonal affective disorder. Side effects noted in recent studies were associated with short term use of St. John's Wort were mild stomach upset, allergic skin reactions, restlessness, sexual/erectile dysfunction, dizziness, dry mouth, and tiredness. St. John's Wort should also not taken with certain drugs,medications,and alcohol as it may interact and be potentially harmful. Also note that the supplement "iron" blocks the absorption of St. John's Wort. St. John's Wort is a relatively safe herb that's been used by many successfully for generations,but caution is always still advised when it comes to use of herb's.

Vitamin B6 (*Pyridoxine*) – Mainly responsible for the production and metabolism of neurotransmitters, serotonin, melatonin, dopamine, norepinephrine, and gaba. Vitamin B6 is responsible for the processing of amino acid's and proteins. It can be found naturally in a variety of foods including red meats,poultry,fish,eggs,non-citrus foods,and cereals. The optimum intake is yet known but the typical dosage range is 2-20 mgs a day,although in can be purchased in varying dosage's 50 to 100mgs.

Folic Acid & Vitamin C – Play a role in the production of serotonin and transmitting brain chemicals.

Sun Light – Bright sunlight increases the production of serotonin in the body and also bright lights,so spend some time in the sun for the serotonin enhancing effect.

Meditation – this helps the nervous system operate at optimum levels,increasing levels of serotonin and endorphins.

Exercise – one of the best natural ways to increase levels of serotonin and endorphins. Try training vigorously for 45 minutes or putting a physical demand on the body to stimulate the effects of serotonin and endorphins. I'm sure at one time or another everyone has felt the soothing calm effects after exercising, whether it be long distance jogging, running, tennis, weightlifting, or even playing basketball.

Pharmaceutical's and Drug's that Enhance Seratonin Levels

Prozac – (*fluoxetine*)- Is a class of pharmaceutical drug's called selective re-uptake inhibitors (SSRI) that was the first approved (SSRI) drug by The FDA in 1987. Used for major depression, OCD, extreme anxiety, generalized & socialized anxiety disorders, and panic attacks. Prozac was the drug of choice prescribed by many physicians during its marketing introduction hype in main stream medicine. Prozac works by adjusting serotonin levels in the brain by preventing the re-uptake of serotonin by nerve cells after its been released.

Since uptake is an important mechanism for removing released neurotransmitters and terminating their actions on adjacent nerves,the reduced uptake then increases free serotonin levels to stimulate nerve cells in the brain. The side effects that have been reported of Prozac are sexual dysfunction in both man and women patients, low sex drive, dry mouth, anger issues, decreased appetite, and headaches.

Paxil (*Paroxitine*) – an antidepressant that's listed as a serotonin re-uptake inhibitor that affects brain chemicals that may be unbalanced. Paxil is also used to similar situations as Prozac and also may be used for additional purposes such as severe premenstrual disorder, premature ejaculation in men and nerve problems that are associated with diabetic neuropathy.

Paxil just as in all (SSRI's) drugs should be used with caution and should not be mixed with any other drugs or medicine's

Lithium – an element that's found in trace amounts in virtually all rocks. Lithiun works with other elements in the brain by increasing serotonin release and decreasing serotonin receptors in the hypothalamus. Lithium is currently the most commonly used drug to treat bi-polar disorders. It serves as a mood stabilizer and is helpful in 70% to 80 % in bipolar patients.

Zoloft - (*Sertraline HCI*) also belongs to a class of drugs called (SSRI's) serotonin re-uptake inhibitors that's used in OCD, panic disorders, anxiety, major depression, post traumatic stress disorder, and premenstrual dysphoric disorder. Side effects are the same as with other (SSRI's) class drugs,low sex drive,sexual dysfunction,etc.

These are just some of the pharmaceutical drugs currently out pertaining to serotonin re-uptake inhibitors,there many more which basically cover what I've mentioned and all pertain to same common emotional disorder's listed in the previous pages. Some people do well on certain listed drug's,and for some people it's a matter of trial and error to see what work's. You have to remember that we are all biologically the same. But sometimes the same drug will have different effects on certain individuals.

The sexual dysfunction's that some of these serotonin drugs may cause will have a different affect opposite of what's mostly commonly experienced,and this is why scientist's today still regard the brain as very complex and not yet fully understood.

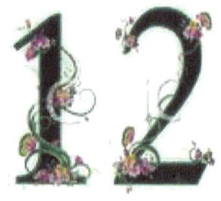

CHAPTER TWELVE

<u>Acetylcholine and Sexuality</u>

Acetylcholine another neurotransmitter in the brain was one of the first to be discovered back in the 1900's. It is involved in memory function, learning,and muscle stimulation that is made from the precursor nutrient "choline" and studies have shown that increasing dietary choline levels can increase the production of Acetylcholine.

In the central nervous system Acetylcholine plays the role in attention and arousal. This neurotransmitter triggers the sexual response in both men and women and with too little Acetylcholine, sexual activity goes down. While not as powerful as dopamine in terms of sexual desire,it is related to sexual arousal and helps to get that "lets get that going feeling" to initiate sex or when the urge strikes you to want to have sex.

As an important neurotransmitter, Acetylcholine when in high decent levels prep's the brain for optimal functioning when it comes to memory, learning and task's at hand. Acetylcholine is also the main neurotransmitter in the parasympathetic nervous system that controls things like heart rate and digestion. High levels of Acetylcholine also make it necessary for you to keep the excitement going in your creativity,marriage,and your desire's. On the opposite spectrum,low levels of acetylcholine can make life very difficult and problematic,like signs of Alzhiemer's disorder, MS, dry skin, dementia, forgetfulness, slow reaction time, unhappiness for no apparent reason, unable to concentrate and focus, and low levels in Acetylcholine may cause vaginal dryness in women,and erection problems in men,non initiation in sexual response, etc., the list goes on and you can begin to see the picture on the importance of optimum levels of Acetylcholine.

Natural Ways to Increase Your Acetylcholine Levels Through Diet & Supplements

Foods that Increase Acetylcholine

- *Egg Yolks*
- *Beef Liver*
- *Chicken Liver*
- *Wheat Germ*
- *Pork*
- *Peanut Butter*
- *Almonds*
- *Oat Bran*
- *Soy Protein*
- *Skim Milk*
- *Shrimp*
- *Lean Ground Beef*
- *Cod, Salmon, & Tilapia*
- *Broccoli*

- ***Trimmed Ham***

- ***Brussel Sprouts***

- ***Cucumber***

- ***Zucchini***

- ***Lettuce***

- ***Ice Cream***

- ***Butter***

- ***Cheese***

- ***Yogurt***

- ***Dried Apricots***

- ***Figs***

- ***Raisins***

Please note that there are many more food choices that are high in choline the precursor to Acetylcholine. The ones listed are basically a much richer source of choline. With the fatty foods being the best. Eggs being the richest source supplies the body with the most choline,125 mgs. With the yolk being the highest.

Supplements That Help Increase Acetylcholine Levels

Supplements may be the easiest way of increasing levels of Acetylcholine

and the fastest.

Choline – An immediate precursor to Acetylcholine that's usually grouped with the B-Complex vitamins and can be purchased in supplement form in many health food stores and pharmacies. The recommended daily intake of choline has not yet been established,but generally for adults dosage's range400-to-500mgs.Choline is relatively safe and side effects are minimal when taken in the recommended dosage's.

GPC-Choline - This is the best absorbed form of choline that exists in your cell membranes and the most expensive form to buy. Dosages range from 500 mgs to 2,000 mgs broken up in two divided dosages taken with meals with breakfast and dinner.

Phosphatidylcholine – Commonly called also as lecithin, is another form that has its benefits as a source of choline and Acetylcholine production. Sold also in granules,liquid,gel caps,and capsules. Dosage is taken as directed by the manufacturer.

Phosphatidylserine – Another component of choline that's very effective and therapeutic that helps increase levels of Acetylcholine. Dosages of 500mgs to 2,000mgs may be broken up in two daily dose's.

Vitamin B5 (*Pantothenic Acid*) – This vitamin assists in the synthesis of choline for the production of Acetylcholine and often used in the above supplements for the production of Acetylcholine.

The Following Supplements Help To Preserve Acetylcholine in The Brain

Manganese – This mineral helps preserve levels of acetylcholine in the brain. Take 1mg to 5 mgs with food daily.

Acetyl-L-Carnitine – an excellent supplement that's been heavily researched and proven very safe, effective, and made popular by anti aging enthusiast. Having fantastic potential in cognitive function and well being. Taken by many health advocates for it's anti aging benefits, brain cell death, bodybuilders, etc.. Dosages range from 1,000mgs to 3,000mgs per day. When combined with Alpha Lipoic Acid 100 mgs to 300 mgs you have a powerful synergistic effect that you can actually feel working in a short period of time.

Huperizine - This herbal extract is one of the proven Acetylcholine esterase inhibitor, meaning it prevents the breakdown of Acetylcholine. This particular supplement borders on being a drug for its proven benefits on Alzhiemers patients and considered safe but caution should still be advised. Dose's are 200mcg's in three divided dosages.

Drugs & Smart Nutrients that Increase Acetylcholine Levels

DMAE – (*dimethylaminoethanol*) A smart nutrient that slows the breakdown of choline in the brain as a result more available choline will be turned into Acetylcholine. Also used by anti aging enthusiasts and college students in preparation for exams.

Pyroglutamate – Is also able to increase Acetylcholine levels in the brain by enhancing the production of brain chemicals to cause more Acetylcholine to be made.

Ginkgo Biloba – *a microcirculatory herb thats used extensively in europe*

In Alzhiemer's disorder, dementia, and cognitive disoders. Ginkgo has the ability to stimulate the blood circulation throughout the body and in the brain. Also stimulates the brain's absorption of Acetylcholine and essential lipid's which aids in the production and release of Acetylcholine into the brain. Ginkgo should not be taken if one is on prescription blood thinners and it generally has a safe track record.

Centrophenoxine – used to treat common senile dementia and Alzhiemer's disease. Centrophenoxine increases Acetylcholine production by improving fluid intelligence in the brain.

Huperzia Serrata – Is an Acetylcholinesterase inhibitor which has been used in china for centuries to treat a number of conditions related to cognitive   disorders including malaria and Rheumatic Fever. It readily crosses the blood brain barrier and acts as an Acetylcholine inhibitor.

Galantamine – An anti Alzhiemers drug that can be bought over the counter that's a very popular Acetylcholinesterase that was first developed in Bulgaria in 1959. Galantamine was originally developed to treat Alzhiemers disease and was FDA approved for that purpose.

Studies and research seem to say that these smart drugs and nutrients which improve synaptic plasticity do have the greatest effect on intelligence, focus,and learning. The sexual effects that we're concerned with come into play cause of their ability to improve brain stimulation and neurotransmitter functioning. Anything that basically affects the brain in a positive manner will to some degree effect sexual function. Of all the brain chemicals in the brain a loss of Acetylcholine is the easiest to notice that something is wrong. You will begin to notice that you may not be initiating sexual response's as you once did easily before your romantic side will be fading slowly and as a man reaction will be harder to maintain. Your cognitive function will also fade, memory, concentration, and learning skills will be impaired.

As with any supplement or drug we should be concerned with side effects and should be taken seriously by researching the supplement or drug at hand,before taking on any supplement regime to better your sexual capacity.

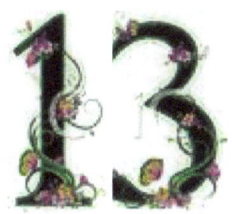

CHAPTER THIRTEEN

<u>Natural Ways to Increase Gaba Levels in The Brain</u>
(*Brain's Braking System*)

Gaba (*gama aminobutyric acid*) A brain chemical that helps to control the brain's and body's pace on a communication basis between the brain and the body. Also an important chemical within the brain. Ggaba is an inhibitory neurotransmitter that serves the brain by the regulation of the firing of neurons.

More than half of the population have a problem with Gaba deficiency. Without it our minds would never stop racing and our muscles would be in a constant stressed situation. Our overall ability to function as a whole would be impaired. Gaba is produced within the brain and has many functions such as HGH production, induces sleep and relaxation, reduces stress and anxiety,and promotes well being in a calm state.

Unlike Dopamine and Acetylcholine, Gaba and Serotonin are the brain's "off" circuits functioning as an electrical switch turning off our sexual desires. They do this by inhibiting communication within brain cells that help regulate or slow down certain bodily process's such as relaxing, sleep, and regrouping by not letting the brain over react to certain situations or stimuli.

With high levels of Gaba people tend to become too committed for many of reasons and then sexuality starts to fade away for you to become restless and anxiety ridden. But by balancing brain levels of Gaba and boosting the other neurotransmitter's, you will then become more in tune and turned on by sex. You will also have a lot more desire for sexual encounters. Just remember that when Gaba levels become unbalanced you will also become unbalanced.

As you can see how unbalanced levels of Gaba have on our sexuality and personal lives, anxiety settles in and then we become stressed which then takes precedence over our sex lives. Cortisol then takes dominance over our body and mind as we learned earlier in preceding chapters.

Natural Foods and Supplements That Increase Gaba Levels

- **Brown Rice**
- **Bananas**
- **Broccoli**
- **Whole Grains**
- **Potatoes**
- **Spinach**
- **Halibut**
- **Beef Liver**
- **Other Organ Meats**
- **Rice Bran**
- **Lentils**
- **Green Tea (very good)**
- **Complex Carbohydrates (high in glutamine)**
- **Citrus Fruits**

- **Walnuts**

- **Korean Kimchi**

You can enhance your own Gaba levels through foods, supplements, meditation (yoga) and exercise stimulation. Which will help with the balance of other neurotransmitters such as, Dopamine, Acetylcholine,and Serotonin. As this book pertains to sex we must note that sex begins in the brain. If our moods and thoughts are not correct one will not be in the mood or right frame of mind to act on any sexual impulses. A healthy brain begets a healthy and satisfying sex life.

Glutamine – An Amino Acid that's the immediate precursor to Gaba. Your body creates Gaba from the Glutamine in your body. There is also more Glutamine in your body than the other 19 amino acids,and through its role in maintaining Gaba levels in the brain it also plays an important role in brain function.

L-Theanine – An amino acid that helps boost Gaba brain levels,that cross's the blood brain barrier very easily. Green tea is also rich in L-Theanine and is often used as a mild relaxation beverage.

Inositol – a vitamin in the B-Complex family that's also related to Gaba that helps to activate brain Gaba levels, Inositol helps you feel calm and relaxed.

Yoga - In itself a form of exercise and meditation is a very positive way of increasing Gaba brain levels as well as increasing or balancing body's hormones.

Taurine - An amino acid that helps increase Gaba levels in the brain and used to treat high blood pressure problems, alcoholism and gall bladder problems.

Valerian - Herbal extract that's used to treat anxiety attacks, and sleep disorders. Valerian helps to inhibit Gaba breakdown in the brain.

Xanax - A popular anti-anxiety drug that's widely prescribed and addicted to many of the young crowd in society today. Xanax works on the Gaba neurotransmitter receptor slowing down the release of norepinephrine and Dopamine. Xanax will also inhibit or slow down sexual desires and more likely be a cause of sexual dysfunction.

Klonopin – A popular and often prescribed by doctors ,functions basically the same as Xanax but for some may work better or less than Xanax. This too will often inhibit sexual desire.

Gaba – An Amino Acid Supplement that can be bought over the counter to help balance and replenish Gaba brain levels in the brain. In higher dosages Gaba also helps with the production of growth hormone. Used for anxiety attacks, addiction problems, mood stalization, and by bodybuilder's for GH (*growth hormone*) production.

These are basically some of the ways of which brain Gaba levels can be increased and of how Gaba affects our sex life and daily moods. As you can see how brain neurotransmitters, Dopamine, Acetylcholine, Serotonin, and Gaba govern the brain's chemistry on sexual behavior.

Each one of these neurotransmitters depends on a balance ,so a deficiency in one neurotransmitter will cause an unblance in the other. A decrease in sexualality may be the first indication that there is something wrong and the brain is not working at its peak levels and producing the right amounts of brain chemicals.

Basically the four components of sexuality can be broken down into phases that correlate to each neurotransmitter such as desire, arousal, and orgasm's.

Too much Dopamine in the brain and you'll have – lots of libido and sex drive. Too little dopamine and you have lack of sexual interest and drive.

Too much Acetylcholine in the brain and you will – feel romantic and with women (*men*) lubricate easily during foreplay. Too little Acetylcholine and you will be dry (*women*) and be unable to achieve an orgasm as easily before and be able to sustain a romantic relationship.

When you have too much Gaba you create too much tension and anxiety and mood for sex doesn't exist. When you have too little Gaba you will feel too uncontrollable for your mate or partner.

Too much Serotonin you won't be able to attain an orgasm as once before and with too little Serotonin your prone to premature ejaculation and women may feel a lack of desire or intimacy.

Each one of your brain chemicals affect the way each one works.

As an example when Dopamine levels are high serotonin levels are low,and by balancing Gaba it will lower Dopamine levels. Through diet, food, exercise and with the help of certain supplements we can maintain a positive and healthy outlook towards our sexuality.

In this book you have the means to understand the basic functioning of brain neurotransmitters and apply what you've learned here in an informed manner. As I always advocate, when in doubt always seek the help of a qualified nutritionist, holistic health practitioner, or your current medical doctor.

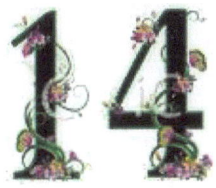

CHAPTER FOURTEEN

Hormonal Sexual Chemistry -Testosterone,Estrogen,and Progesterone

Hormones are chemicals produced by glands in our body that the brain transfers and regulates as it interprets its chemical signal from the various organs and glands. Hormones basically are produced from cholesterol that is vital to our health. Usually produced in the liver from the foods we eat and if too much is produced we collect a waxy substance know as plaque.

Plaque as we know creates a disorder known as arteriosclerosis that impairs blood flow to our heart and vital organs and glans,and if not corrected can lead to heart attacks and premature death. The result of this leads to sexual dysfunction,and in men erectile dysfunction,cause of the lack of blood flow to the male penis. It is now known that erectile dysfunction may be an early warning to heart disease.

Testosterone

It is estimated that here in America over 5 million men suffer a condition called Hypogonadism or low testosterone while other men simply have low testosterone because of aging and type of lifestyle.

Signs of low testosterone are low libido in men and possibly women. A decline in well being, moods, & lack of desire in certain tasks, depressed moods, easily irritated, sleeping problems, loose skin, decreased beard growth and hair growth, loss of vitality, and inability to maintain an erection.

In men Andropause typically begins around the age 40, but it can occur early if under constant stress and the abuse of drugs, alcohol, reckless life style and poor eating habits. Some of the sexual symptoms of early Andropause include lack of sexual desire and arousal, premature ejaculation, a lack of intensity in orgasms, erectile dysfunction, decreased size in penis length and scrotum.

Testosterone is synthesized from Androstenedione a by product of DHEA and Progesterone. Although we think of Testoeterone as a male hormone. Women also produce small amounts of Testosterone as well and have receptors in their nipples, clitoris, and vagina, enhancing sensitivity to sexual pleasure and stimulation.

Many women will experience a variety of sexual and physical symptoms when their testosterone levels drop too low. Testosterone deficiency in women will manifest itself as low libido or sexual urge, impaired sexual function that at times approaches itself as complete aversion to sex. It also affects their emotional sense of well being, loss of bone mass, muscle tone, and strength.

Testosterone being the main hormone that basically controls sexual libido in both men and women,but in women small amounts are also produced in their ovaries and adrenal glands. While some Testosterone can also be produced from Progesterone and DHEA hormones in both sexes.

In males testosterone is responsible for maintenance of sex drive -

–	Growth of the penis,testes, prostate gland, and scrotum.

–	Deepening of the voice.

–	Maintenance of hair growth and body fat.

–	Production of sperm.

–	Erectile function,and hardness of the penis.

–	And some research also leads us to believe that it reduces male risk of heart disease.

Also not that most of the testosterone circulating in the blood stream gets bound to a protein called sex hormone binding globulin (SHBG) ,and the remaining testosterone that's left around 5% total or less is the most active form. When symptoms such as low libido or sex drive occurs despite normal levels of circulating testosterone,this may be due to circulating levels of   Testosterone becoming bound to sex hormone binding globulin – (SHBG) making Testosterone less available and active.

Fortunately there are things that one can due to free up the available testosterone and make it more active to rev up our libido and sexual desire.

This will be covered in the next following chapter concerning natural foods and supplementation.

Natural Supplements To Help Increase Testosterone

Foods that help increase essential fatty acid intake and Prostaglandins will actually help to increase one's sexuality. Essential fatty acid's are needed by the body,brain,nervous system,and all the vital organs and glands which are necessary to every cell in our body. They are the precursors of hormone-like substances called Prostaglandins which are important for sexual response.

The two essential fatty acids that we need in our diet from food are Omega-3's, Alpha Linolecic Acid and Alpha Linolenic Omega-6. CLA or conjugated Linolecic Acid Omega-6 may increase the production of Prostaglandin E1, that increases brain levels of the hormone Somatotropin. This hormone increases the output of growth hormone(GH) which in turn increases Testosterone.

When both sexes are deficient in essential fatty acids,we experience the following in men insufficient ejaculate during intercourse, infertility, low sperm count, slow recovery, and tire easily. In women infertility, vaginal dryness, and PMS symptoms. When essential fatty acid levels are optimum,we tire less easily,and feel more sexually active with increased energy levels.

Flax Seed Oil - Helps enhance testosterone levels in the body by supply polyunsaturated Omega-3 fatty acids and Lingans,it also helps to control estrogen levels in men which boosts Testosterone. Flax Seed Oil comes in gel capsules, granules, and in liquid form. Taking 2 tablespoons of flax oil two times a day and before bed will help boost your Testosterone levels.

Fish Oils - Good source of Omega-3 fatty acids that help the body also to boost testosterone and help clear the circulatory system of unhealthy fats that clog our blood vessels.

Sweet Potatoes/Yams – natural source of testosterone that is rich in natural sterols, diosgenin, which when extracted in labs produces the hormone progesterone.

Massularia Acuminata – A western African native plant that has been used for food and medicine that contains natural steroid-like chemicals that are similar to Testosterone. Massularia has a reputation for being a libido booster,and a study in Nigeria showed that the plant boosts natural testosterone by as much as 60% in subjects being tested. Massularia Acuminata is popular among avid weightlifters and bodybuilders. It can be purchased on the internet or in a health food store that sells a good line of herbal products.

Garlic – A very therapeutic cure-all that's used in kitchens around the world is a very good testosterone producing food and supplement. Allicin the main medicinal component of garlic is the active ingredient. Scientific studies have also proven it to decrease cortisol and raise testosterone levels. Also helpful in circulatory stimulation which benefits the body in many healthy ways,such as lowering cholesterol,raising HDL levels,immune system enhancement,and besides it taste's good too ! This is one food/supplement to pay attention to,make sure that when you purchase it in supplement form that its extracted for its Allicin content.

Zinc – is needed by both men & women but in men the requirement is abit more substantial,meaning it benefits the prostate gland,sperm production,testosterone levels,fertility,and should be taken with B6 and magnesium to aid in zinc absorption and in the free conversion of chlesterol to testosterone.

Tribulus Terristis – one the best and popular herbal supplements that raise testosterone levels in an indirect way by elevating the hormone Leutenizing
Hormone (LH) which stimulates the production of testosterone in

the testes. Once made popular by Eastern European Olympic athletes stating that it helped their performance. The active components of tribulus are two steroidal compounds, Furostanol Glycosides and Spirostanol Glycosides. When purchasing make sure its extracted in the standardized form of Protodioscins, preferably the highest percentage possible. Tribulus should be taken on a course of 4 weeks on and 2 weeks off,and can be repeated after a break.

Horny Goat Weed – (*HGW*) - Another very popular and effective herb that seems to not only boost testosterone but also elevate nitric oxide levels as well that dialate the blood vessels to greatly increase blood flow to your vital
genital region. It has been used in Chinese medicine for hundred of years for its sexual stimulating affects in both men and women. This herb also inhibits the enzyme PDE-5 ,making it an PDE-5 inhibitor like Viagra and Cialis. Icarrin is the active ingredient responsible for the sexual effects of this herbal extract. When purchasing make sure you find the highest percentage of Icarrin available.

Tongkat Ali -(*Eurycoma Lonifolia*) -This herb comes from the island of sumatra where it is the only place left to harvest. Primarily used as an aphrodisiac and erectile dysfunction amongst the native's in Sumatra and the rest of the world. It too has been made very popular among the bodybuilding crowd for its ability to greatly increase testosterone levels four fold DHEA, and IGF-1.Tongkat Ali does have other medicinal values beside its Testosterone boosting affect such as Anti-Malaria, fevers, high blood pressure, fatigue, and anti-aging affect.
Our concern and what this book is about sexual enhancement, Tongkat Ali will help restore a lagging libido and erectile dysfunction is what we're most intersted in. Tongkat Ali comes in an extract potency just make sure it's the Sumatran brand and look for the highest extraction possible for the most beneficial effect.

Tongkat Ali should be taken daily as it requires time for the testosterone levels to build up in the blood. The extracts should be cycled on a two to one basis for the best result. For example take the product for two weeks on and one week off before using again for two weeks. You may also take it for four weeks on and two weeks off,and for some people they made to increase or lower the dosage as usage amounts vary do to body weight and height.

Nettle Root Extract – (*Urtica Dioica***)** nettle root has been documented as a nourishing herb that strengthens all systems of the ***body. Traditionally*** nettle has been used to treat arthritis, tuberculosis, hay fever, coughs,and allergies. What we're concerned with is its sexual enhancing effect, in which it does very well. Nettle will help with impotency,hence its effect on prostate problems,and it ability to free up free testosterone.

The active ingredient 3, 4, Divanillyltetrahydrofuran should in its extract form with the highest percentage of standardized extract available for its greatest effect. For men, nettle frees up free testosterone and prevents it from being converted (aromatized) into Estrogen.Too much estrogen plays havoc on a man's sex life by binding to receptor sites that contribute an over production of sex hormone binding globulin (SHBG). Sex hormone binding globulin binds free testosterone in a way that makes testosterone unavailable to receptor sites in the brain, nerves, and genitals.

Some studies show that the decline in sexual interest with advanced age is caused by the binding of testosterone to globulin by the SHBG. This explains why some men on Testosterone replacement therapy do not respond to testosterone .

Royal Jelly – A bee by-product that contains hormone like substances that support glandular and reproductive function. It is also the only natural source of pure Acetylcholine,which we learned earlier about in previous chapters. Royal jelly has been shown to be a very active substance and therapeutic,involved in the conduction of nerve and sexual impulses. When taken it can support stress levels and boost Testosterone levels, increase's sperm count and mobility,and increase energy levels. Just make sure that the royal jelly you buy comes in a creamy like paste and its kept cold that's the real royal jelly. For some people its effects are noticiable within days,their moods and well being improves,stamina increases,and sex life is much more satisfying.

DHEA- (*dehydroepiandrostene*) also known as Androstenolone,is an important endogenous steroid hormone that is the most abundant circulating hormone in the body. It is produced in the adrenal glands,brain,and gonads where it functions predominantly as an androgen in men and an estrogen sex steroid in women.

DHEA production peaks in the mid 20's and steadily declines as we age,and known to be a bio-marker in the aging factor. Being a precursor to male and female sex hormones, DHEA has been found to increase a flagging sex drive in both men and women. It also claimed to have a number of astonishing benificial effects from regulating the immune system,improving physical and emotional well being, decreasing body fat levels, lifting low moods, enhancing memory and mental clarity, reducing stress, regulating sugar control, reducing the risk of impotence,and possibly extending life span. Before taking DHEA,it is best to have your levels tested through either a blood test or a saliva test to see if you need supplementation. Dhea requirements vary from person to person and it is important not to take too much especially if your a women, as it can have masculine effects and unwanted hair growth. Dosages vary ,for low sex drive it is usual to start with a low dose of 5mgs – 10 mgs and you may increase if it is ineffective up to a dose of 25mgs.

Velvet Deer Antler – a very potent source of hormones,minerals,amino acids and enzymes as well as cartilage. Velvet antlers contain both the male and female hormone precursors. High levels of Leutenizing hormone (LH) have been found in the antler extracts that stimulate testosterone production. Velvet antler also helps produce IGF-1 levels that has become very popular with the bodybuilder's in local gyms.A very good supplement to add your arsenal of testosterone producing supplements. Note that not all velvet antler extracts are of high potency,as many fly by night companies are getting on the antler bandwagon and being accused of under dosing their products. One company that has been producing the velvet extract is www.nutronicslabs.com and can be bought on the internet. The supplements are the ones that I think would do the most justice to your cause,there are many more and I can go on forever listing them.

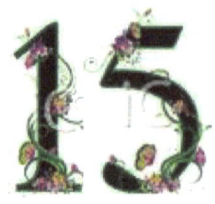

CHAPTER FIFTEEN

<u>Estrogen Cause & Effect</u>

Estrogen, a predominate female hormone that affects every organ system in the body -brain,reproductive system,cardiovascular,and bones. Not only is it a predominate female hormone. Men do need it as well only in smaller amounts.

Women have three kinds of estrogen hormones – estrone, estradiol, estriol, with estradiol being the most abundant of the three. Follicule-stimulating-hormone (FSH) and leutenizing hormone stimulates the production of estrogen in the ovaries. Some smaller amounts of estrogen are also produced in the adrenal glands, liver, and in the breasts.

As women age the predominate hormone estrogen slows down,while estrone
and estradiol increases. When the ovaries lose their functioning in producing estrogen during menopause, estrone then becomes the primary estrogen. Some of the common signs of estrogen withdrawl are,poor vaginal lubrication,loss of libido,depression,bad moods,and hot flashes. As estrogen levels fall so does the neurotransmitter serotonin affecting our moods and behavoir.

Menopuase, typically speaking can be a downer for some when it pertains to their sex life,especially when they once were active for only it to become difficult and avoidable for some women. Symptoms such as vaginal dryness,itching,burning,and some women get UTI's from bacteria that's transmitted during intercourse because their vagina's are too dry.

Fortunately there are things that we can do to restore and balance hormaonal health,through food,diet,and supplements. In the next chapter we will go through a list of foods and supplements that will help balance estrogen levels.

Foods & Natural Supplements That Help To Balance Estrogen Levels

Increasing soy and fish consumption is a healthy way of restoring levels of estrogen and combating sexual dysfunction. It is interesting that Asian women experience less menopausal symptoms than women in America do. Part of the reason is that their diet is centered around heavy soy and fish consumption.

Fish and fish oils are loaded with essential fatty acids that can help the body replenish vital hormones and amino acids necessary for a healthy sex life and well being. Soy products contain Phytoestrogens that have both Estrogen and Progesterone like compounds,which is why foods like fish and soy are important to our hormonal health.

- *Salmon*
- *Tuna*
- *Mackeral*
- *Sunflower Seeds*
- *Alfalfa Sprouts*
- *Flax Seed Oil*
- *Whole Grains*
- *Yams*
- *Nuts-(All)*
- *Pumpkin*

Evening Primrose Oil, Borage Oil, Black Currant Oil – All contain Gamma Linoliec Acid that help with the production of Estrogens in the body. A good combination of the three can be found in certain formulas that provide a synergistic effect.

Boron – This mineral may help increase the body's levels of estrogen and testosterone in women which may lead to a heightened increase in sexual desire. Boron can be bought in health food stores and through the internet.

Maca - This herb from south America is said to be one of the best herbal supplements that help replace natural estrogen levels in a women's body. Maca is considered a vegetable,similar to the turnip that grows in the Andean plateaus of Peru. Considered a food in Peru and has been noted for its libido enhancing affect in women and also in men.

A highly nutritious super food, Maca is loaded with minerals,enzymes,amino acids,and hormone precursors. It is increasingly becoming very popular for its sexual stimulating effect and the balancing of hormone function, Maca has been prized by the local natives in Peru since the Incan Empire. Note that also the Peruvian government has invested a lot in its scientific research to show of its libido enhancing affect of this herb. Here is a list of benefits that Maca can supply the body with in both men and women.

The Amazing Qualities of Maca -

Massive increase in Sexual Function

Decreases Impotence and Erectile Dysfunction

Improves Hormonal Imbalance & Testosterone Levels

Increases the Production of Sperm Cells

Elevates Moods & Depression

Increases Energy, Stamina, and Vitality

Regulate Women's Hormonal Imbalances

Helps reduce Menopausal Symptoms in Women

Regulates Women's Menstrual Irregularities

Ease's PMS Symptoms

Reduces Male Andropause Symptoms
There are no negative side effects with maca use, and is considered safe. This is one herb that I have personally used and found it to be very helpful and useful.

Kacip Fatimah – (*Labisia Pothoina*) may be one of the most sought after female tonics and aphrodisiac in the world. Grown in the Malaysian rainforest, Kacip Fatimah has been used for many generations by women in malaysia to induce and facilitate childbirth. It is also well know for its other amazing benefits too numerous to mention, but for its libido enhancing effect is what we're conserned with.

For its sexual enhancing effect Kacip Fatimah acts as an Estrogen receptor modulator (SERM) like the drugs Tamoxifen or Raloxifene. Through this process, Kacip Fatimah increases free levels of testosterone from the ovaries producing the sexual stimulation effect often seen when taken this herb.This herb is not a relatively easy herb to find and purchase,however there some sites on the internet that do list it. See www.BarlowesHerbalElixers.com.

Solutions To Sexual Problems & Herbal Aphrodiciac's

Popular Supplements for:

Impotence & Erectile Dysfunction– **Herbs***;Tribulus Terrestis, Tongkat Ali, Dodder Seed Extract, Korean Ginseng, Bulbine Natalensis, Maca Extract, Black Ant Extract, Butea Superba, Horny Goat Weed, Cnidium Monneri Extract, Xanthoparmelia Extract, Cordyceps Extract;* **Amino Acid's** *-L-Arginine,L-Citrulline;* **Bee Products** *– Pure Royal Jelly (paste)*

Low Libido & Lack of Desire -Herb's;Tongkat Ali, Tribulus Terrestis, Maca Extract, Horny Goat Weed ,Catuaba Bark Extract(women), Clavo HuascaExtract(women), Kacip Fatimah(women), Damiana Extract(women);Amino Acid's,L-Phenylaline(women), PEA(women),Mucuna Puriens Extract(men/women),

Tetosterone Enhancer's – Herb's;Tongkat Ali(men), Kacip Fatimah(women), Tribulus Terrestis(men), Horny Goat Weed(men), Dooder Seed Extract(men), Korean Ginseng(men), Maca Extract(men/women), Cordyceps Extract(men), **Bee Products***;Pure Royal Jelly(men/women).*

Premature Ejaculation – herbs;*Dodder Seed Extract, Cnidium Monneri, Xanthoparmelia, Butea Superba, Black Ant Extract.*

Vaginal Dryness/Lack of Lubrication – *essential fatty acids, Omega-3's,Fish Oils, Flax Seed Oil, DHEA, Pregnenlone, Royal Jelly.*

Note; by following the tips and suggestions in this book you have the means of turning your sexuality into a most rewarding endeavor. Also,it always pays to do your own research on any supplement,herb,or product that you are considering to try. I encourage you to take responsibility for your own personal health and education and to seek out reference material's on sexual health and vitality.

Disclaimer

The suggestions in this book are not to replace the care and supervision of a professional health care Physician. If you are taking any prescribed medications for any pre-existing medical matter,it is advised to seek the approval of your primary health care physician.

The information presented in this book is merely for informational purposes and should be taken as such.

www.ingramcontent.com/pod-product-compliance
Lightning Source LLC
Chambersburg PA
CBHW041502280526
45792CB00004B/1105

* 9 7 8 1 4 7 7 6 7 6 7 7 6 *